Military Diet

Lose 10 Pounds in 3 Days

Disclaimer

While the author has taken utmost efforts to ensure the accuracy of the written content, all readers are advised to follow the information mentioned herein at their own risk. The author cannot be held responsible for any personal or commercial damage caused by misinterpretation of the information in this eBook.

All information, ideas and guidelines presented here are for educational purposes only and readers are encouraged to seek professional advice when needed.

The quest for slim, fit bodies is a never-ending journey fraught with innumerable challenges. If you are one of those looking for easy-to-implement fitness routines that deliver guaranteed results, you have come to the right platform!

The Military Diet is one of the more recent fitness regimes that emphasize on the chemical makeup of foods you consume to limit your calorie intake and therefore shed those extra pounds off the weighing scale. Contained in here you will find:

1. A brief introduction to different diet regimes
2. A detailed analysis of why such regimes do not work
3. An in-depth explanation of what the Military Diet is and how it works
4. A list of things included in the Military Diet
5. A list of things prohibited in the Military Diet
6. And much more!

So if you really want to get rid of the extra fat in your body, come and experience the Military Diet plan with us. This eBook contains all information pertaining to the Military Diet plan that you need to know before diving into it.

So what are you waiting for? Get your copy today! It is up for grabs!

Contents

Disclaimer 2

Introduction 5

Defining Weight Loss 6

Diet and Exercise Go Hand-in-Hand 8

Why is it Difficult to Lose Weight? 11

Contained in Here 13

Military Diet Plan 14

What is So Different About it? 15

What Does it Entail? 19

The Special Military Diet Rule 20

Diet and Exercise to Go Hand-in-Hand 20

The Daily Schedule 21

DAY 1 22

DAY 2 25

DAY 3 28

The Next Four Days 31

Healthy Suggestions 31

The Underlying Principle 46

What Does it Curtail? 48

Conclusion 51

Introduction

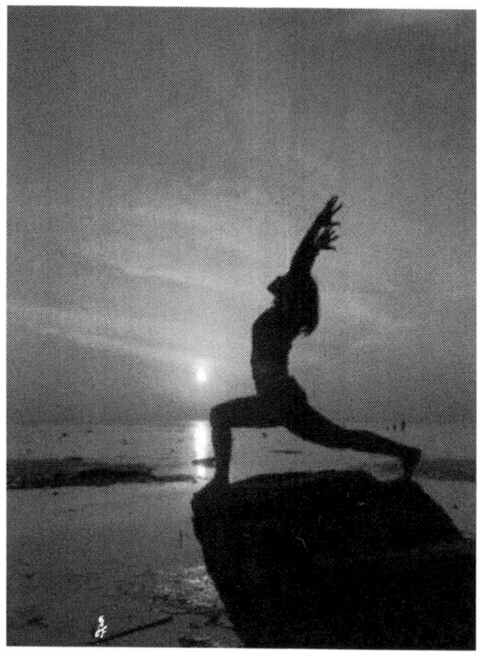

For males as well as for females, looking good is one of the fundamentals of feeling good. Physique matters a lot whether it is about fitting into a dress and looking good wearing it or about attracting people's attention and enjoying the stares you get while showing off a brilliantly toned body. Even though it seems to be a mutually shared dream across the masses, very few are lucky enough to turn these figments of imagination into reality.

There are several dozens of fitness regimes formulated and promoted by people from all walks of life – it is no longer specific to nutritionists or fitness experts. With the increasing numbers of "fitness solutions," the numbers of disappointed customers are also on the rise.

Most of these miraculous solutions fail to deliver their promises and are eventually led into obsolescence. Just a handful of these are adequately equipped to deliver what they advocate!

It is not only about the apparent inches and the superficial pounds but also about the inherent balance of your body that plays a role in defining your fitness level. Most people are misled into believing the former is all that they seek only to discover they end up worse off than when they started. For this reason we believe the definition of weight loss and fitness is in order. So here it goes!

Defining Weight Loss

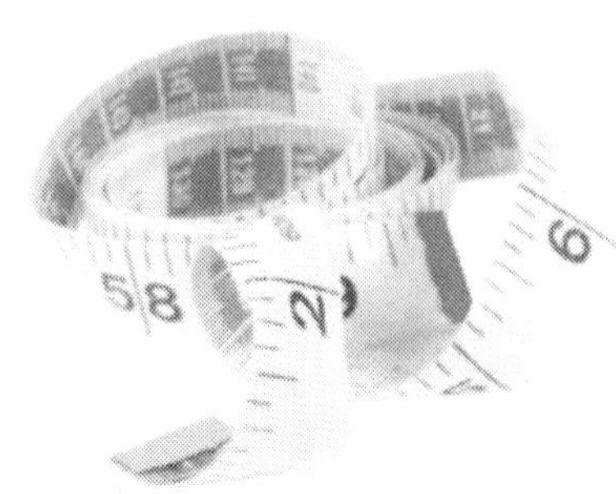

Typically, most people think fitness is all about shedding off the extra fat content in your body so that the inches shrink automatically. Little or no attention is given to the fact that your health does not depend on these inches, (at least not directly) but is rather dependent on internal body balance.

The idea behind attaining fitness is to achieve the correct internal body balance which does not only translate into enhanced strength, balance, stamina and well-being, but also promotes longevity. The goals and results have a long-term focus as compared to the short-term focus most people have these days.

If you've achieved your dream physique but at the same time tend to remain ill often, the purpose and motivation of your fitness is lost. Same is the case if you experience unexplained fatigue, lethargy and negativity.

Fitness is a positive notion and should therefore not be associated with negative emotions. If you don't feel good about your fitness goals or achievements, it is most probably because you are not doing it right!

There are two fundamentals that define your health. Firstly, it is the food that you consume. Secondly, it is about how you put this food to use.

Whatever you eat becomes a part of you in innumerable ways. It provides energy for you to be able to perform your functions and duties – internally and superficially. If you are consuming more than you are using up, you are eventually storing up the balance between the two. When it is the other way around, your body creates a deficiency and ensures that it is felt. This is how the natural body mechanism works.

Your body has a built-in balance correcting mechanism which comes into action immediately as an imbalance is felt. Whether it is the overflow of nutrients or deficiency thereof, your body treats both conditions in the same way. So you end up feeling as though something is not right. This is precisely the point when you need to rethink your fitness regime.

Weight loss is not just about getting the extra pounds off your weighing scale or the inches off your body; it is about feeling at your best internally as well as externally. Contrary to popular belief, the former benchmarks fail to incorporate essential elements. So even if you attain your objectives, you subconsciously pave the way for bigger problems.

Diet and Exercise Go Hand-in-Hand

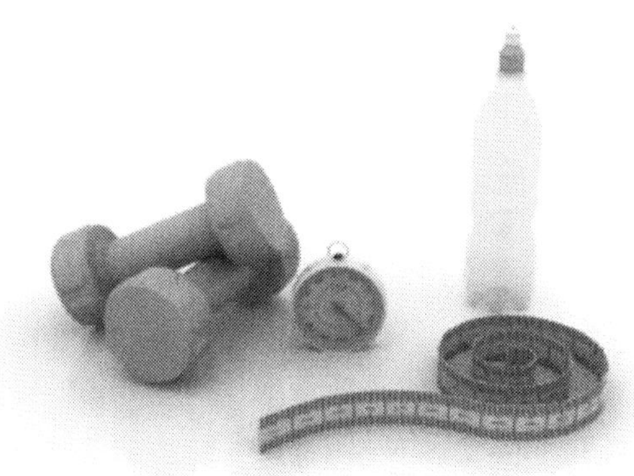

Diet and exercise go hand-in-hand. It is not possible to achieve your fitness goals while focusing on any one aspect of your health. They are components of a continuous cycle that governs your course of life.

Whatever you consume is disintegrated into constituent particles and absorbed into your body through the complex mechanism of digestion. Once absorbed, these nutrients are put to several different uses including repair of worn-out tissues, neutralization of body balance, and replenishment of body's energy reserves and so on and so forth.

The food you consume is made up of several million unique nutrients that serve a specific purpose. There are no foods that offer the perfect combination of all nutrients in the right quantities to provide for your daily nutritional needs. Consequently, you need to consume several different types and kinds of food to meet your daily requirements.

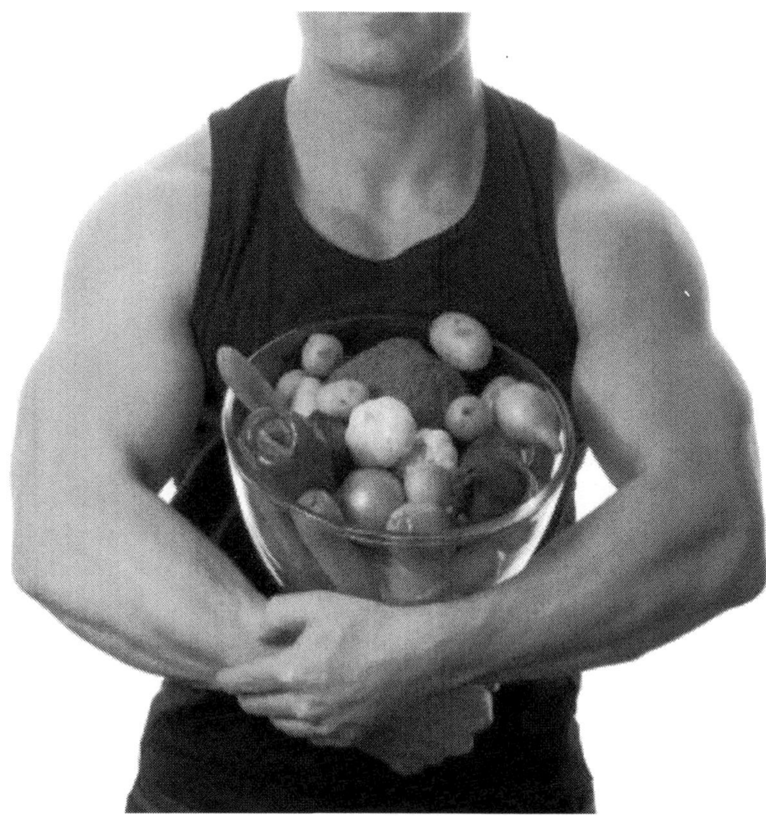

In doing so, it is possible for you to mistake a good combination of foods to be synonymous with healthy foods. Consuming multiple foods does not mean you should be eating relentlessly. On the same note, it does not mean you over-eat a particular delicacy that you like and eat a little quantity of other foods that are known to contain important nutrients but do not agree with your taste buds in the same way. It is important to strike a balance across all extremes to make sure your motives are being met.

Healthy eating is about consuming the right foods in the right quantities and at the right times. Eating outside the proper meal timings disrupts your natural body cycle. This also means your body is incapable of making use of the food you eat in the right manner. You will feel hungry at odd hours and are therefore more likely not to make healthy eating choices.

The quality and quantity of foods you consume are extremely imperative in defining your health. Eating the right foods does not mean you can transgress on the quantities and, likewise, eating the right quantities does not mean you can eat anything you wish. Both aspects go hand-in-hand to promote overall health and well-being.

And when you have resolved this part of the equation, the next most important thing to figure out is how to use this "food." When this food is absorbed by your body, it performs several million different functions to maintain your bodily functions. A major proportion of your food is transformed into energy. This energy is utilized when you move around and perform different activities. If the reservoir is not depleted completely, the excess is transformed into glucose and fats to be stored in your body.

Needless to say, your fitness regime is incomplete if it focuses only on diet or on exercise. Both aspects go hand-in-hand to promote overall well-being and to help you achieve your fitness motives. The right combination can not only help you decrease the inches and the pounds but also maintain a healthy internal balance so that you feel active and healthy at all times.

So what is it going to be for you – inches, pounds or overall fitness?

Why is it Difficult to Lose Weight?

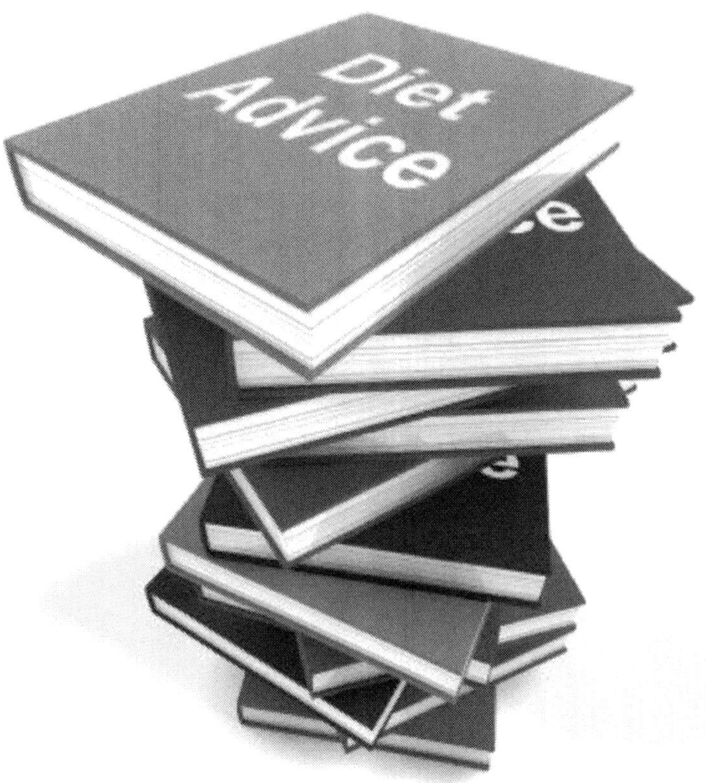

Weight loss has become one of the most difficult tasks to achieve for a number of reasons. The most basic reason for this is that most fitness regimes fail to incorporate the essentials so that the desired results cannot be achieved.

In simple words, most fitness regimes are not doing it right. Most of these tend to be biased about certain aspects of the fitness routine so that the wholesome result becomes impossible to attain. Some diet regimes will focus almost exclusively on your diet while others want you to exercise day in and day out, irrespective of the time constraints you face. The result is not really surprising when such regimens backfire miserably!

A lot has been put into research to find out what works and what doesn't when it comes to weight loss and fitness. While the right way to approach the task at hand is to go through this information before formulating your own recipes of disasters, this is one thing most non-professional experts fail to do. They do what they *think* will work. So even if it does, the results are temporary and fraught with other health challenges.

The bottom line is that everybody is different. The needs for each person in terms of exercise and diet are different. So it is foolish to try putting the same shoe on every foot and expect it to fit perfectly. The stimulants your body responds to may not be as effective for the person next to you. And if this examination is not conducted, the success of the fitness regime cannot be guaranteed.

Staying stringent on your fitness schedule is a colossal task on its own. It requires discipline, will power and motivation to keep doing the same things over only to see meager changes.

It is not possible to transform your body in a jiffy. It requires consistency and perseverance to attain a noticeable difference in you. However, when you fail to see the desired results within the promised time frame, it becomes even more difficult to stay put with the regimen. Not only this, it may even shatter your confidence in other fitness plans so you end up settling for nothing at all!

Simply put, you need a fitness routine that works and delivers the promises it makes. You do not want to be disappointed after being loyal with your routine for a considerably long time period. You need the results to appear readily to keep you motivated and sturdy on your pathway to success.

In other words, you need the Military Diet regime!

Contained in Here

What will you find in here that can benefit you on your way to success? The one word answer is: Everything!

In this eBook, you will find information about everything that you need to know in order to follow the Military Diet plan precisely and to enjoy the results you are hoping to see. From the basics of the military diet plan to its brief history and success stories about those who have been there and done that – this eBook aims to give you a wholesome exposure to the innovative idea of weight loss.

It works and delivers its promises with each passing day. Moreover, it is infinitely different from its competitors so it does not only work, but also keeps you motivated throughout the time period. It gets easier over time so you can reap the fruits of your efforts in a timely manner.

Keep reading to find out everything about a weight loss plan that works! It's all in here so make the most of it!

Military Diet Plan

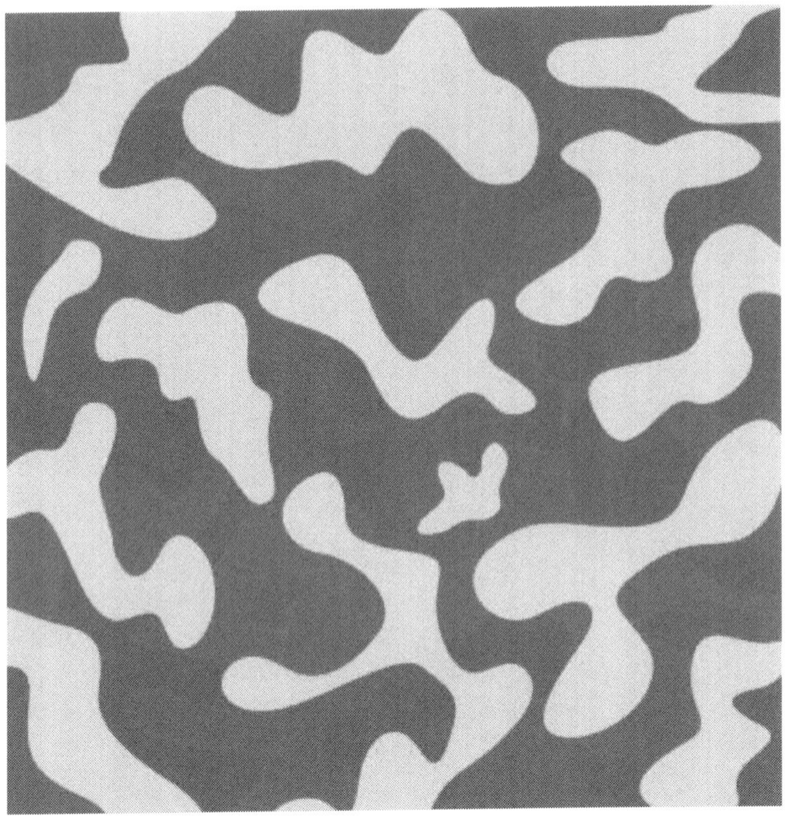

The military is well known for its discipline, its superior strategy-making capabilities and its ability to deliver what it promises. As they guard countries and safeguard every resident that lives inside (irrespective of their nationalities and residential statuses), they symbolize bravery, responsibility and harmony. They are an inspiration for all those hoping to put their lives in order to achieve greater goals.

That being said, the Military Diet also aims to deliver the same. It aims to help you achieve your goals in a disciplined manner that is not only productive but also motivating in itself! Here is a little insight about the military diet regime and how the plan works!

What is so different about it?

If you are thinking this is just another plan in the weight loss puzzle, rest assured this is not the case. The Military Diet plan is built different from the others so that it delivers what others do not!

How is it different from conventional fitness regimes? Here is the answer to all your questions!

1. The Military Diet plan works!

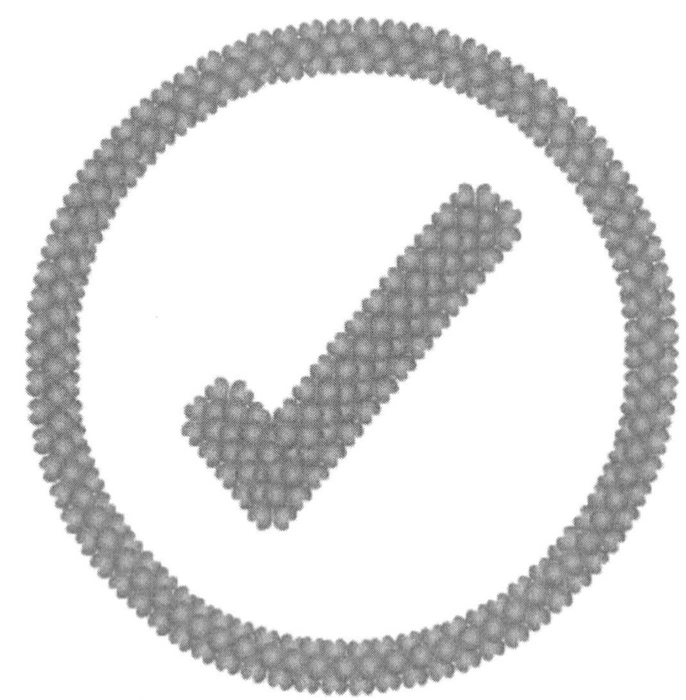

This is the most important distinction the Military Diet has received in contrast with other fitness plans. It works and delivers its promises within the given time frame. The ideology and mechanism is different, which helps you achieve the desired results!

So whoever decides to try the Military Diet plan will definitely be able to achieve his/her fitness goals. In fact there are quite a few success stories circulating around like wildfire! Are you ready to be one of them?!

2. It *incorporates* cheat meals!

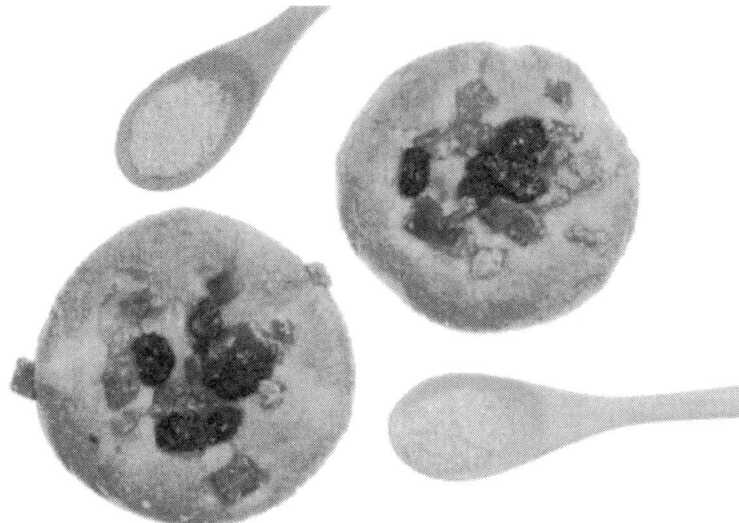

The regime compels you to follow strict diet for three days and then take four days off the diet plan! As wild as it seems, this is how the diet plan works!

In effect, it is almost like following your regular diet with slight changes. It is the three days of work that pays off throughout the week! Could it get any more amazing and wonderful?!

3. The military uses it!!

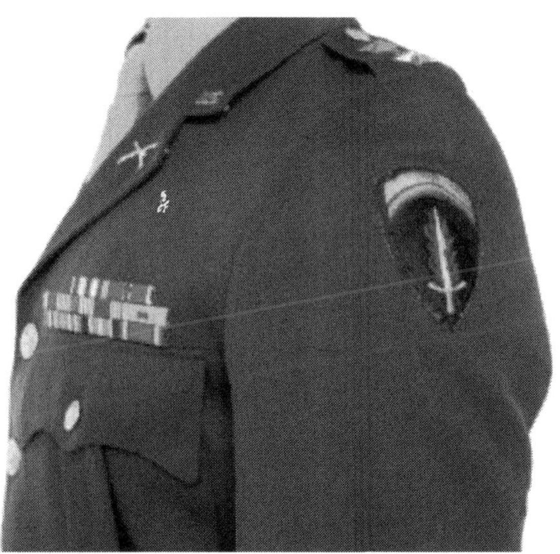

It works for them! What makes you think it will not work for you?!

The diet plan is attributed with the military and this is the way they are able to remain fit and healthy while on their missions. It does not deny you from essential elements of life. It merely suggests altering the way these elements are combined so you can achieve better health and fitness levels!

4. Super quick results!

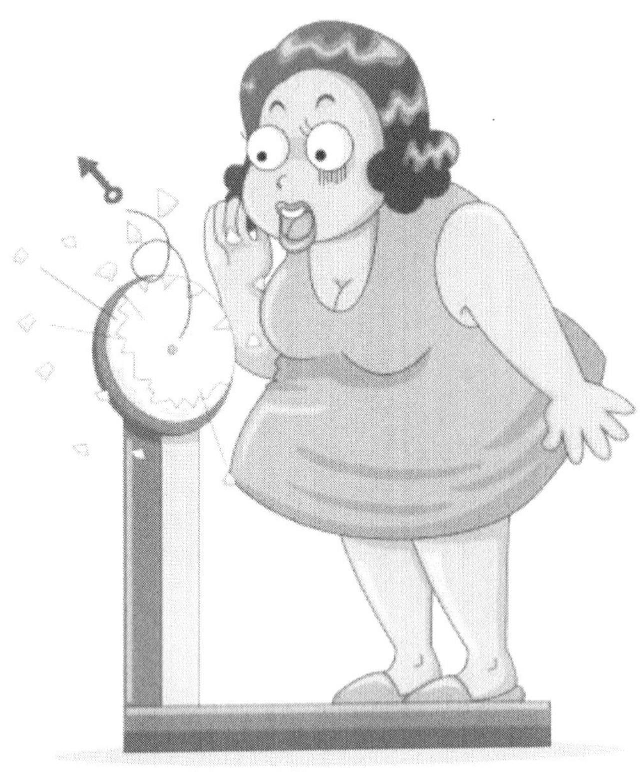

You can lose 10 pounds in 3 days! It sums up to 40 pounds per month! You will begin to witness differences immediately as it yields results quickly.

So whether it is about getting slimmer to fit into a specific dress or to look physically appealing at a special event – the military diet plan is your only rescue that works!

Do you still need more reasons to believe what it can do for you?!

What does it entail?

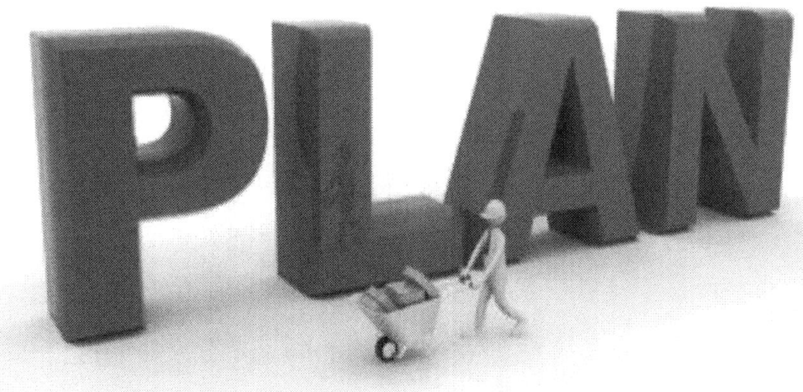

Once you have accepted the fact that Military Diet plan does work, the next important thing is to understand what it asks from you and how it works!

This section covers all aspects of the Military Diet plan in adequate detail to help you achieve overall fitness in less than a month! So are you ready to learn about the miracles of Military Diet plan?

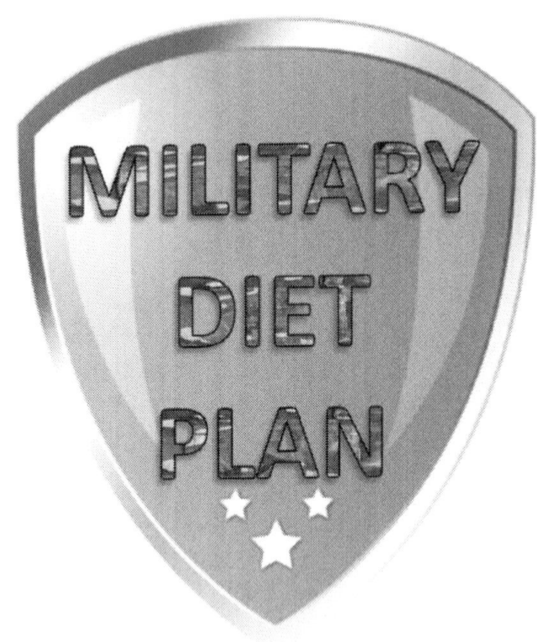

The Special Military Diet Rule

The Military Diet plan compels you to follow a special course of meals for three days and to follow the regular routine then on for four days. There are a few restrictions with respect to the foods you are not allowed to consume – even on off days. The rest is all good!

Diet and Exercise to Go Hand-in-Hand

At this point, it is important to highlight that the Military Diet plan does not intend to work out of the regular. As mentioned previously, diet and exercise go hand-in-hand while helping you achieve your fitness goals. To think that one could work without the other is to hope for a miracle you know will not happen.

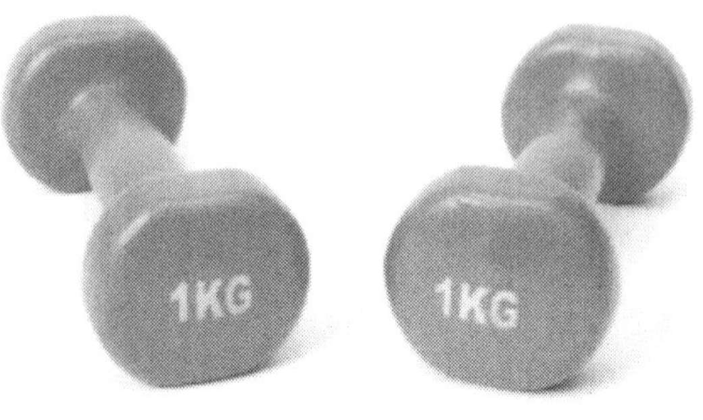

The Military Diet plan is incomplete without exercise. However, there are no specific forms or types of exercises suggested by this scheme. It depends on your personal convenience and availability of time. The idea is to keep some form of exercise in your routine that is focused on your problem areas. Whatever you consume should be put to use before there is a chance for your body to stock it up!

Consult your local gym or fitness expert to find out which forms of exercise will complement the Military Diet regime. Do take time out of your busy schedule to exercise. Once you have got hold of the gist of the Military Diet plan, it will come to you naturally!

The Daily Schedule

The Military Diet plan works for three days and then allows you to take four days off the schedule. Here is what you should be consuming on your three days of the diet. Make sure you follow the given directions closely.

The Military Diet focuses on the chemical composition of the foods. The foods have been selected in such a way that their aggregate affect helps you in losing weight. It triggers the fat-burning mechanism of your body for greater overall fitness.

So while you would be tempted to play around with the diet plan, it is in the best interest of your desired results that you remain stringent with the given regime. And then again, you only need to follow it for three days and then you get to take four days off! What more could you possibly ask for?!

DAY 1

Breakfast: 1 slice of whole wheat bread with 2 tablespoons of peanut butter, 1 cup of caffeinated tea or coffee (without sugar or cream) and ½ grapefruit.

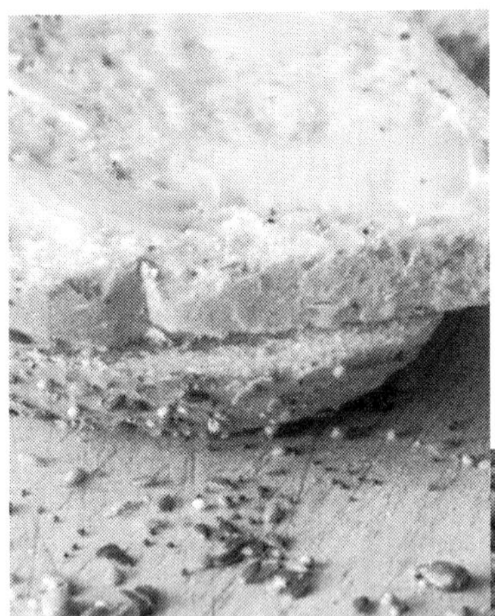

1 slice of toasted whole wheat bread with 2 tablespoon peanut butter

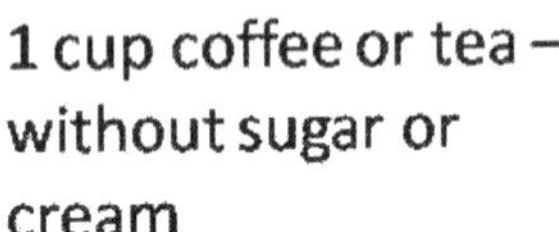

1 cup coffee or tea – without sugar or cream

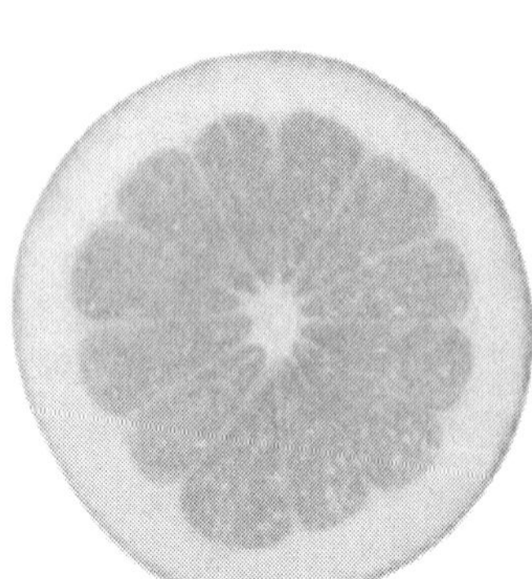

Half a grapefruit

The use of sugars and cream is prohibited for its fat content. It is advised not to use artificial sweeteners either. However, using natural sweeteners like Stevia is allowed.

This marks a healthy start to your day.

Lunch: For lunch, you can have 1 slice of bread either plain or toasted as per your desires, 1 cup coffee or tea without any added sugars or creams and half a cup of tuna fish.

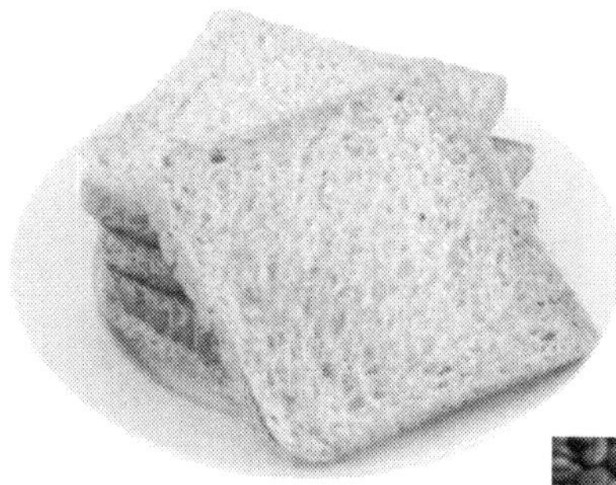

1 slice of toasted or plain whole wheat bread

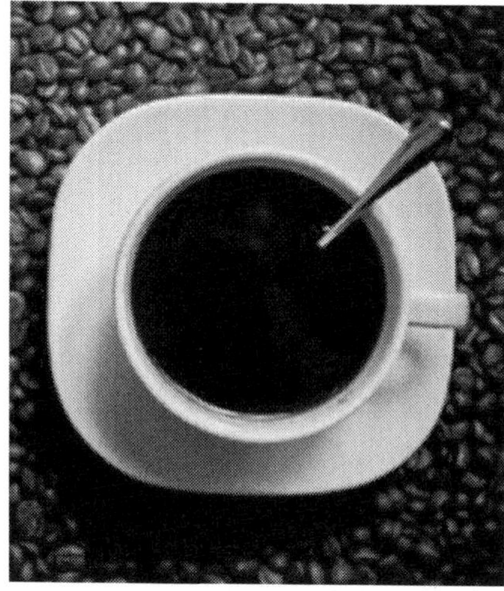

1 cup coffee or tea – without sugar or cream

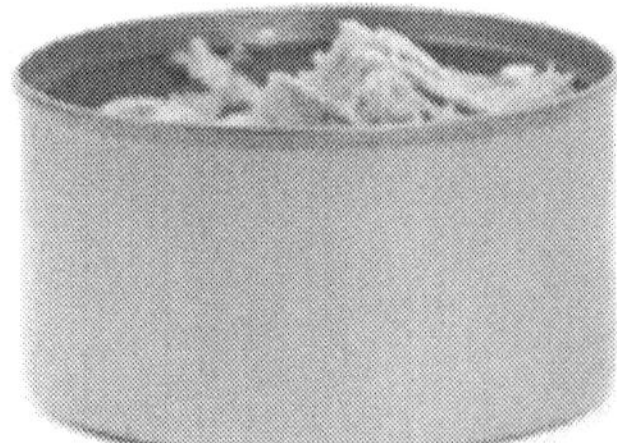

Half cup tuna

This meal provides adequate energy to get you through your daily activities. If you feel exhausted at any point during the day, you can opt for healthy snacks – covered later in this eBook.

Dinner: The last meal of the day has to be magnificent to wind off the day in a sprightly manner. For dinner, you are to consume 3 ounces or about 100 grams of your favorite meat, 1 cup of fresh green beans, 1 small-sized apple, half a banana and 1 cup of vanilla ice cream.

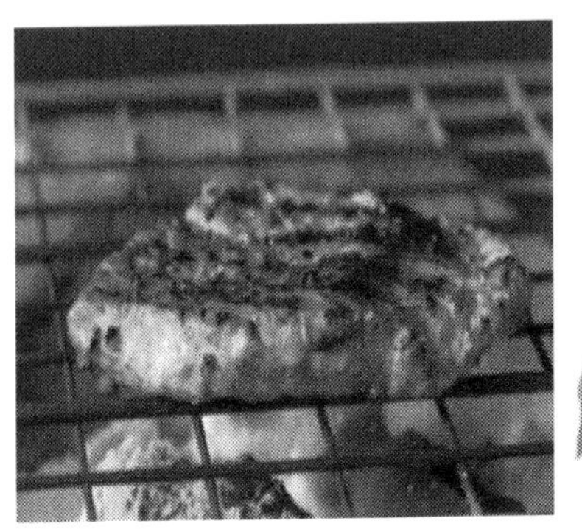

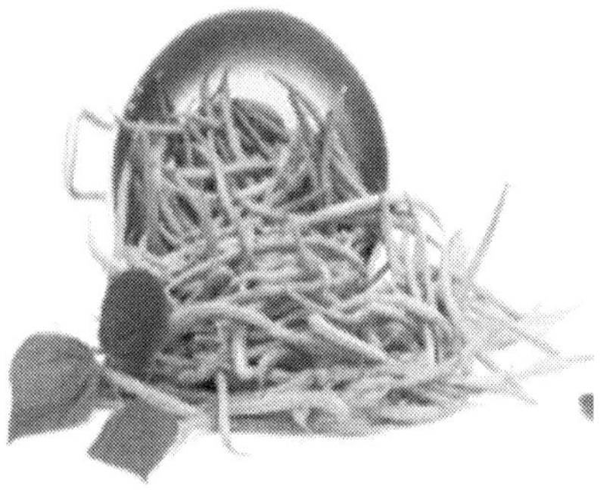

About 100grams of your favorite meat with 1 cup green beans for dinner

For sweet, 1 small apple, half a banana and 1 cup ice cream!

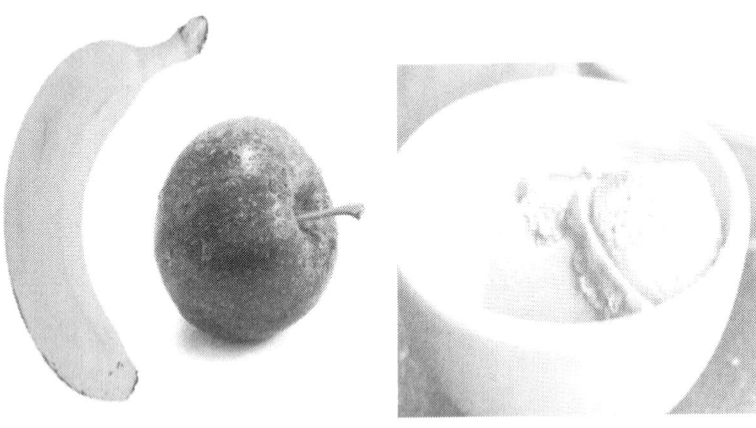

Reward yourself for your effort in following the diet plan with a cup of ice cream. You can also eat other flavors of ice creams – just make sure the sugar content in these is low.

During the night, your body will be able to perform its repair functions normally so you wake up the next day feeling refreshed and revitalized!

Here is what you need to do the next day:

DAY 2

Breakfast: 1 slice of whole wheat bread either toasted or plain, 1 egg cooked in any way you like and half a banana.

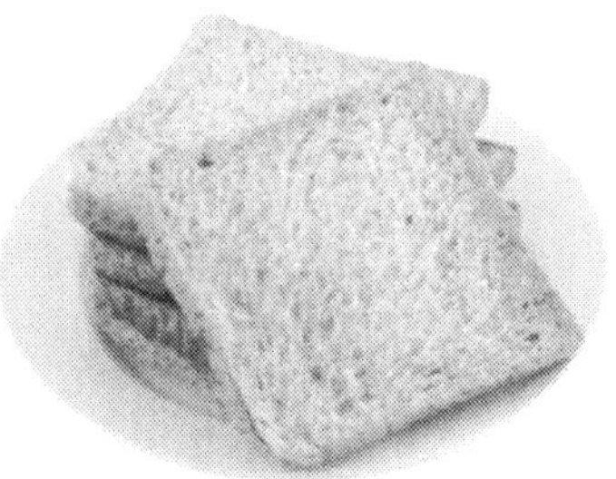

1 slice of toasted or plain whole wheat bread

1 egg cooked in any way you prefer

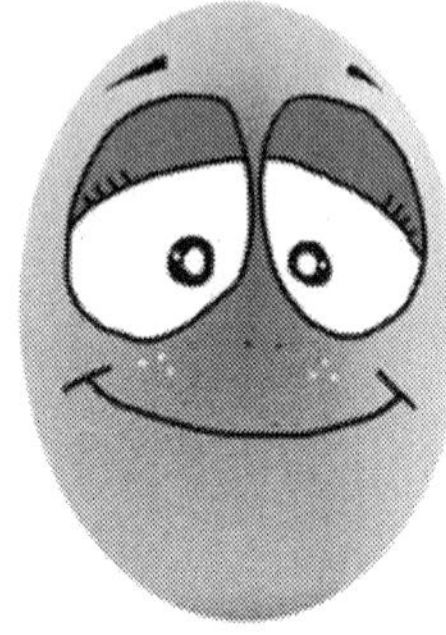

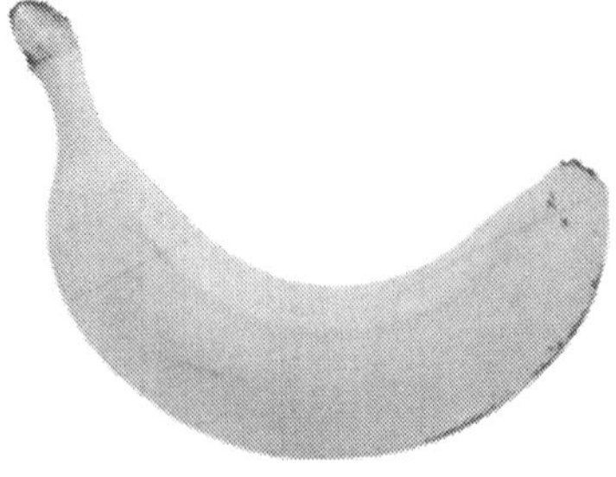

Half a banana

This provides you the energy you need to begin the day with full fervor. Then comes lunch!

Lunch: For lunch, you need 1 hardboiled egg, 1 cup cheddar cheese and 5 saltine crackers.

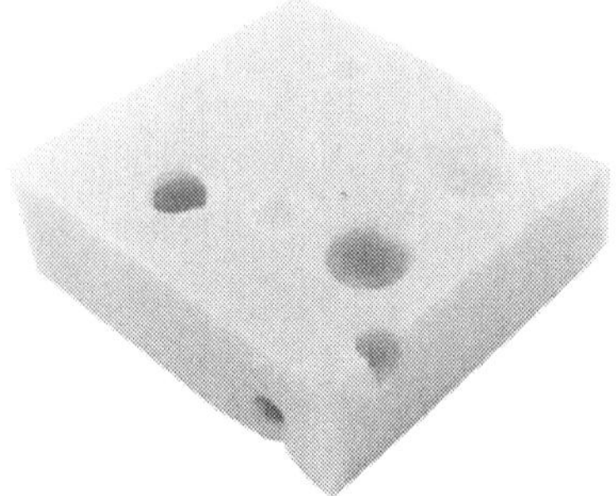

1 cup cheddar cheese

1 hardboiled egg

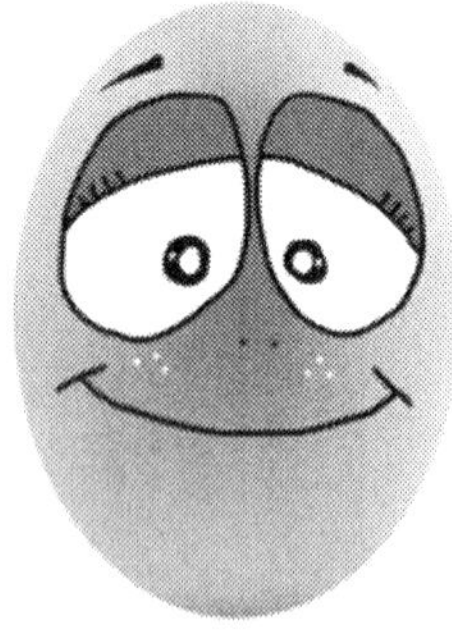

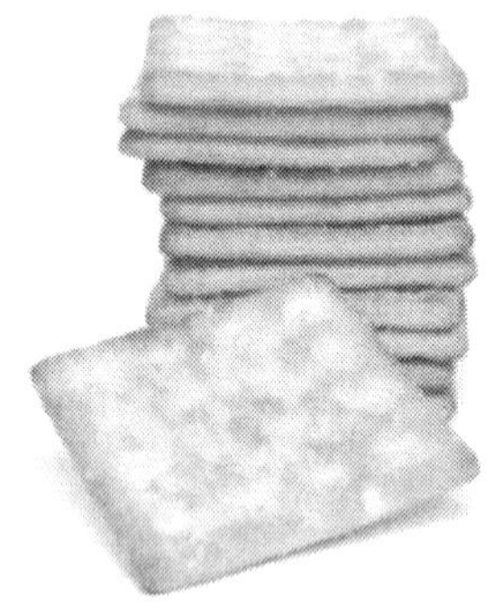

5 saltine crackers

This should be enough to provide for your day's nutritional requirements. Alternatively, you can opt for healthy snacks.

Dinner: For dinner, you'll eat 2 hot dogs without buns, 1 cup of fresh broccoli flowers, ½ cup of fresh carrots cut into your desired shapes, ½ a banana and ½ a cup of vanilla ice cream.

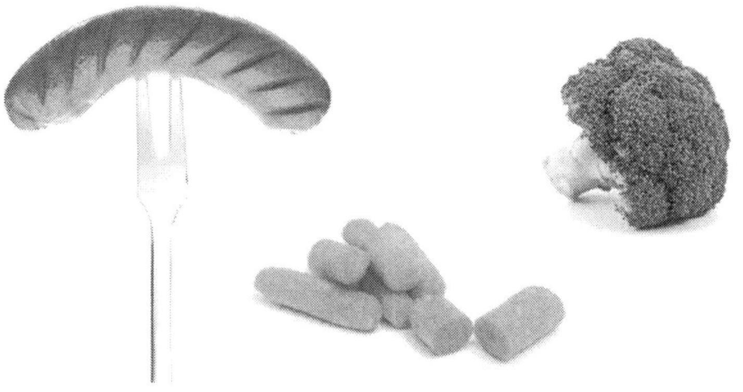

About 100grams of your favorite meat with 1 cup green beans for dinner

For sweet, 1 small apple, half a banana and 1 cup ice cream!

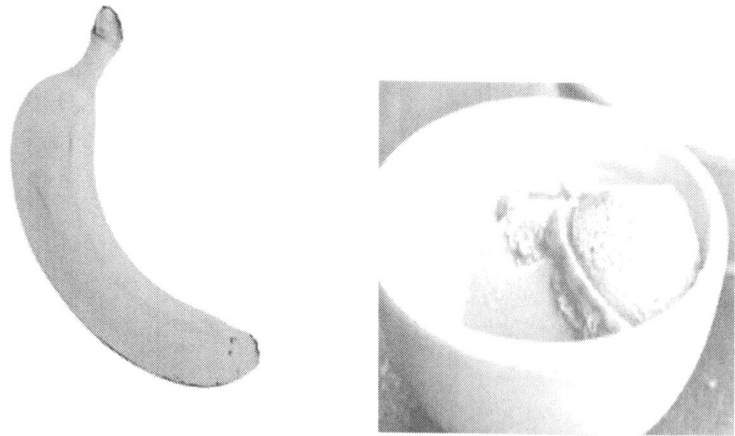

The bowl of ice cream is a sign of reward that you give to yourself after the day's diet. In effect, it keeps you motivated to follow the diet the next day and so on and so forth!

DAY 3

Breakfast: For the third day, you can have breakfast with 1 apple, 1 slice of cheddar cheese and 5 saltine crackers.

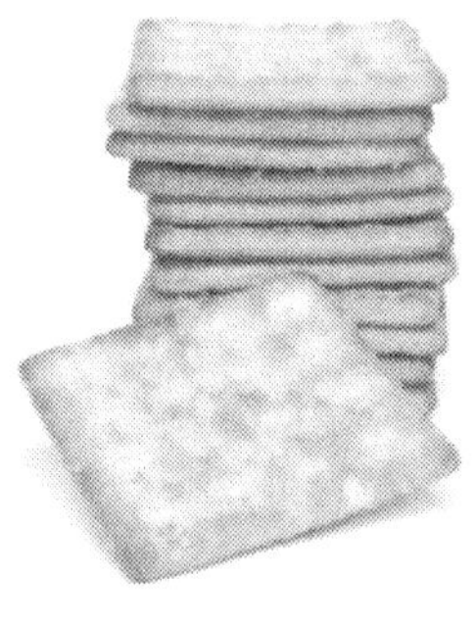

5 saltine crackers

1 slice of cheddar cheese

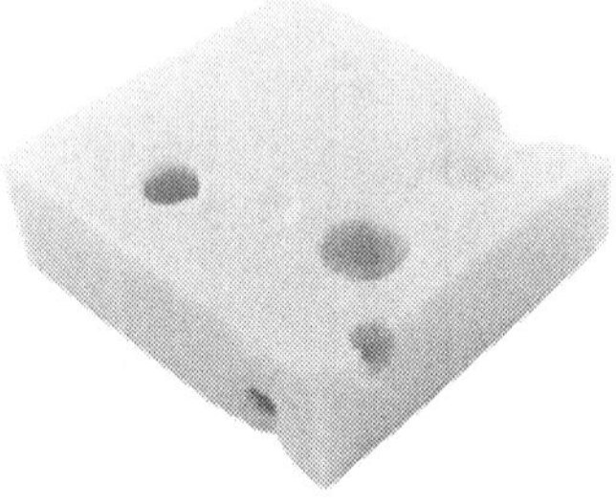

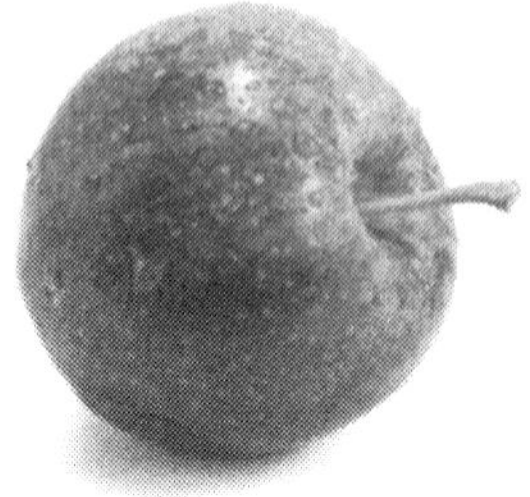

1 small sized apple

This gives you an energy-packed beginning to a fulfilling day ahead!

Lunch: For lunch, you can have 1 slice of whole wheat bread (toasted or not is up to you) and 1 egg cooked according to your desires.

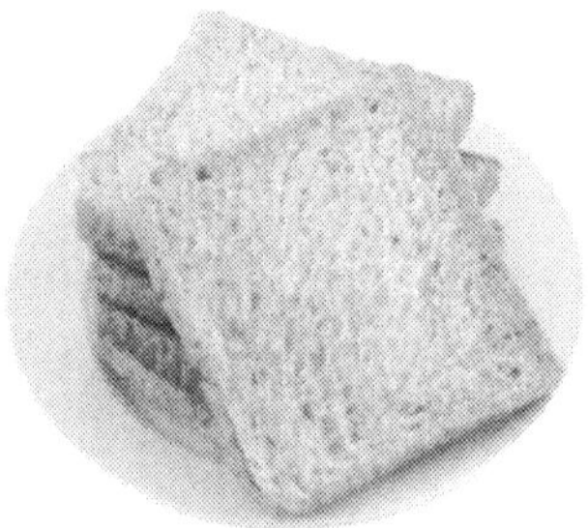

1 slice of toasted or plain whole wheat bread

1 egg cooked in whatever way you like

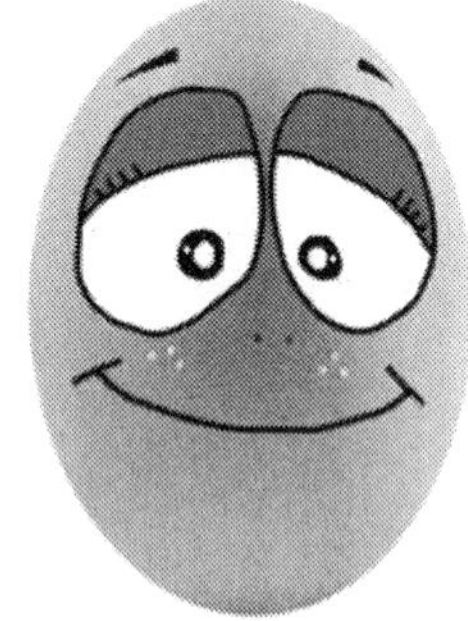

It is advised that you should not deviate from the diet plan mentioned in here. However, if you do, opt for healthy snacks only as they are less likely to hinder your progress towards fitness and weight loss.

Dinner: Dinner for the third day should include 1 cup of tuna, ½ a banana and 1 cup vanilla ice cream.

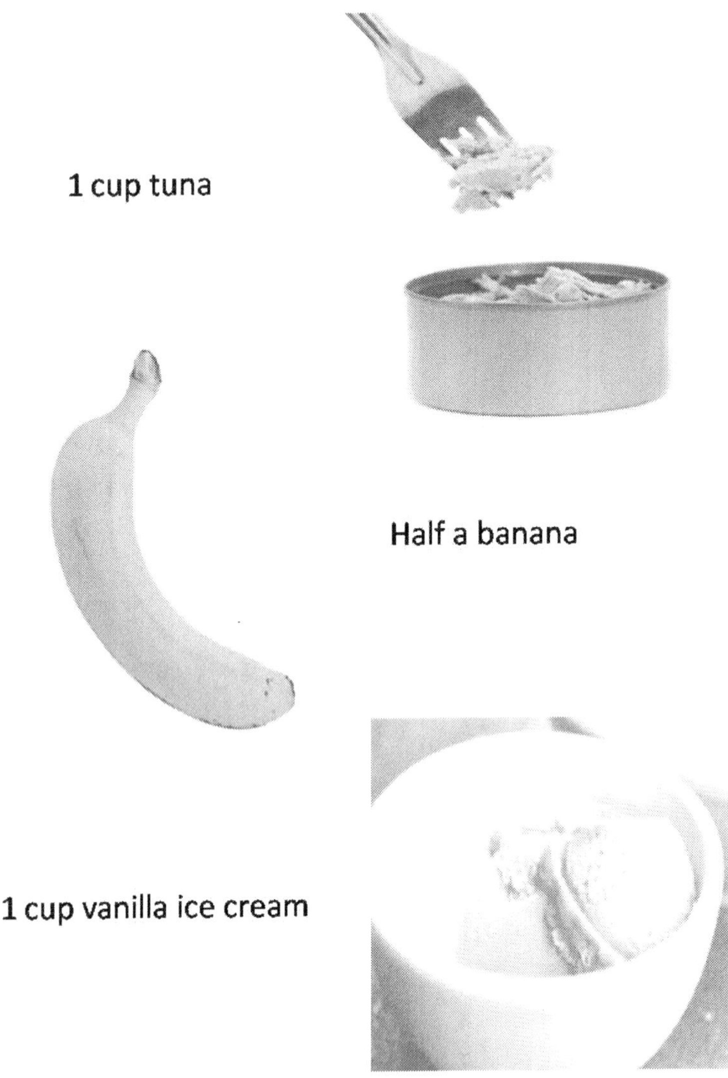
1 cup tuna
Half a banana
1 cup vanilla ice cream

The Next Four Days

Once you've followed the aforementioned diet plan for three consecutive days, it is now time to take a break. For the next four days, you can enjoy regular meals and your favorite delicacies!

There is just one limitation – whatever you consume, it should have a maximum of 1500 calories given your daily calorie usage is more than 1500 calories. You can eat all kinds of foods as long as the total calorie count remains at 1500 calories!

Keep in mind that beverages are also included in this calorie count. So if you are consuming caffeinated tea or coffee without sugar and cream, add 10 calories to your daily consumption. You can mix and match the food items but make sure the aggregate remains the same!

Healthy Suggestions

Here are some of the meal suggestions for the remaining four days of the military diet. Choose whichever suits your taste buds – the rest should be fine!

<u>Breakfast Choices:</u>

Yoghurt with Nuts and Berries: 1 cup yoghurt, 1 cup mixed berries, ¼ cup granola seeds and 1 tablespoon almonds.

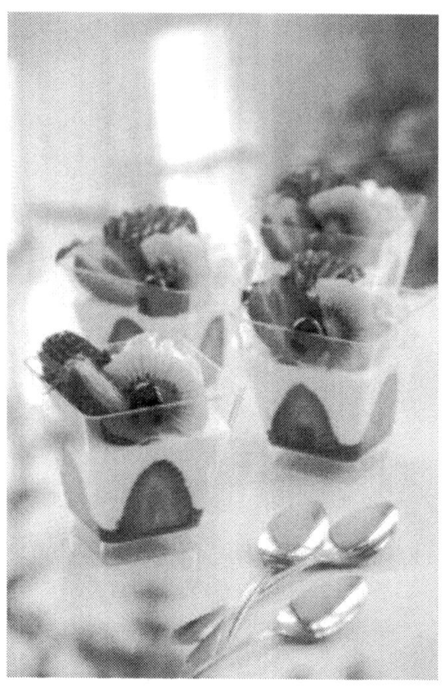

Banana Shake with Citrus Side: 1 cup of milk, 1 banana, 1 cup oats and 1 orange.

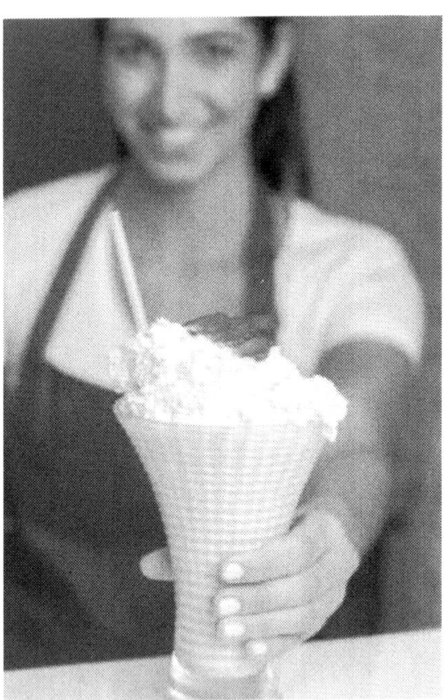

Egg and Toast: 1 egg, 1 teaspoon butter, 1 slice of whole wheat bread, 3 tomato slices and ¼ of avocado sliced.

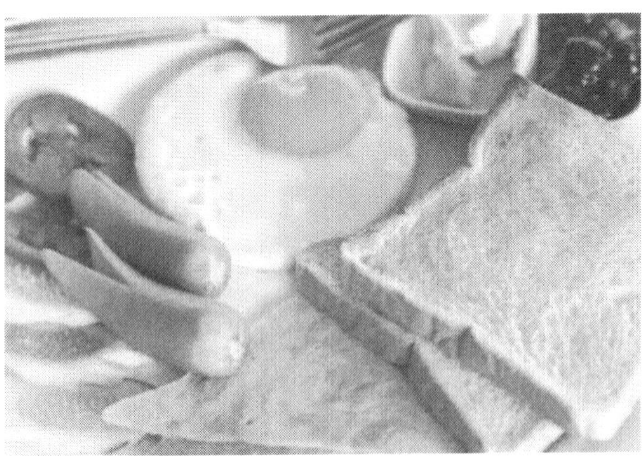

Bread and Fish: ½ whole wheat bagel, 1 tablespoon cream cheese and about 20-gram serving of salmon. You can add tomato slices, cucumber slices and onions if you want.

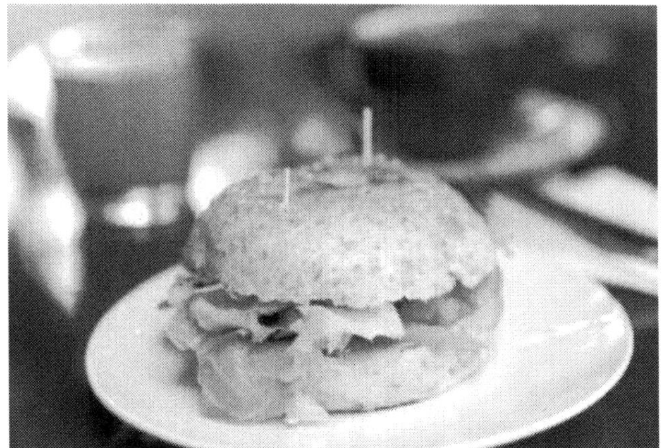

Oatmeal with a Twist: 1/3 cup oats, 2/3 cup milk, ½ cup apple cubes, 2 tablespoons roughly chopped walnuts and cinnamon.

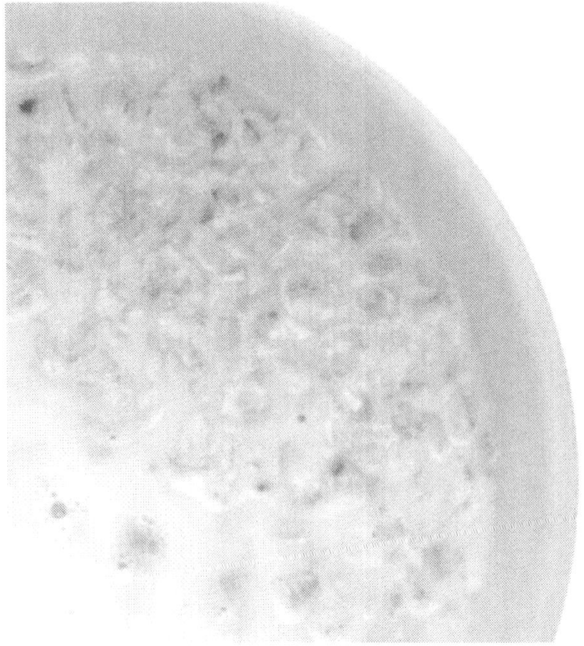

Waffles with Berries and Walnuts: 2 waffles topped with ¼ cup strawberries, ¼ cup blueberries and 7 walnuts.

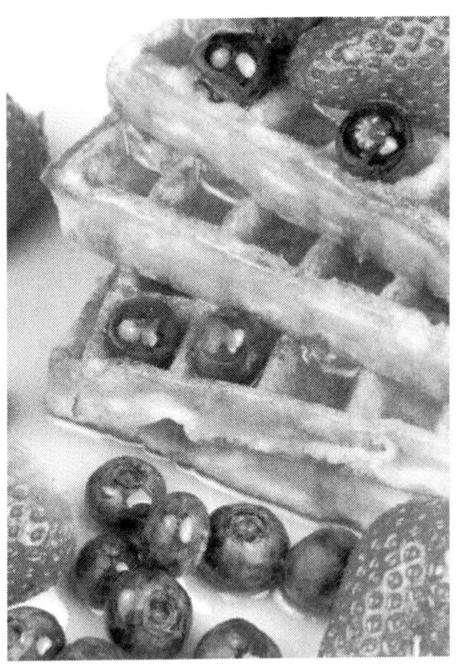

Spinach and Egg Muffin: 2 whole wheat toasted breads topped with 2 eggs (preferably scrambled) and 1 cup cooked spinach.

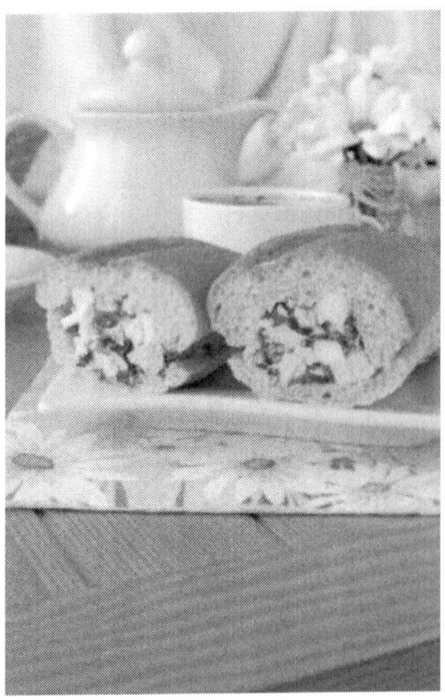

Almond Butter with Pears: 1 slice of whole wheat bread topped with 1 tablespoon almond butter and 1 pear.

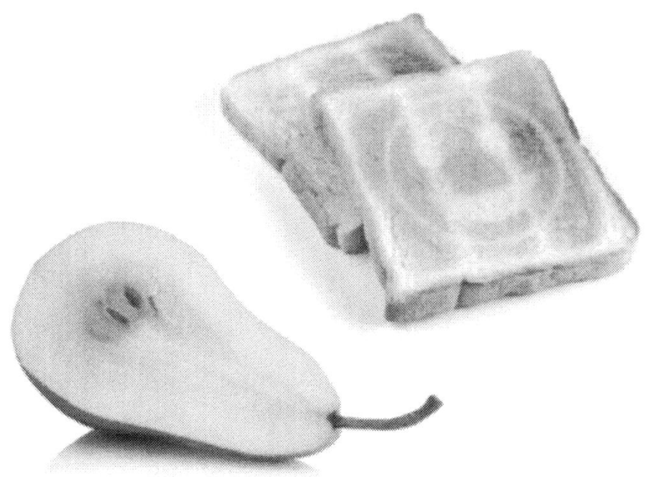

Ricotta Cheese with Tomato and Basil Toast: 1 slice of whole wheat bread topped with 1/3 cup ricotta cheese, 4 tomato slices and a few basil leaves.

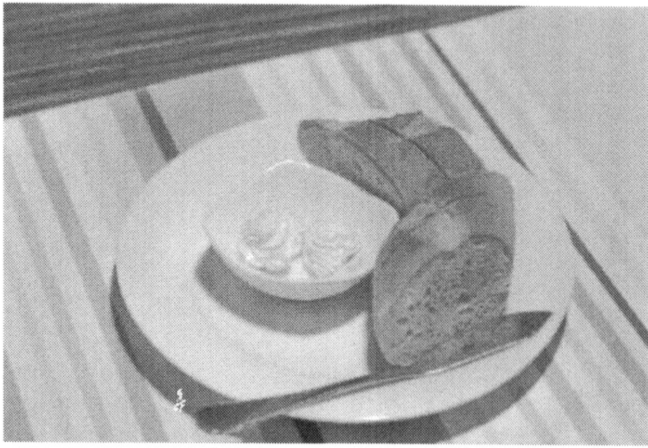

Sweet Banana/Strawberry Shake: 1 cup plain soy milk, 1 banana (you can use an equivalent amount of strawberries as well), 1 tablespoon honey, 1 tablespoon flaxseeds and 2 tablespoons oatmeal.

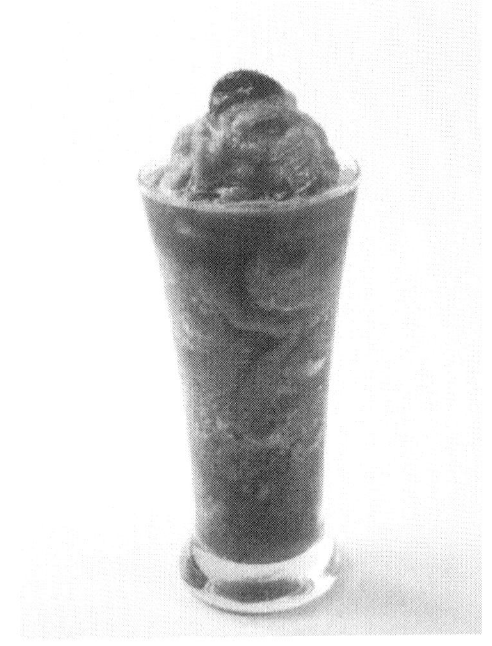

Cheese Omelet: 2 eggs cooked with ¼ cup cheddar cheese.

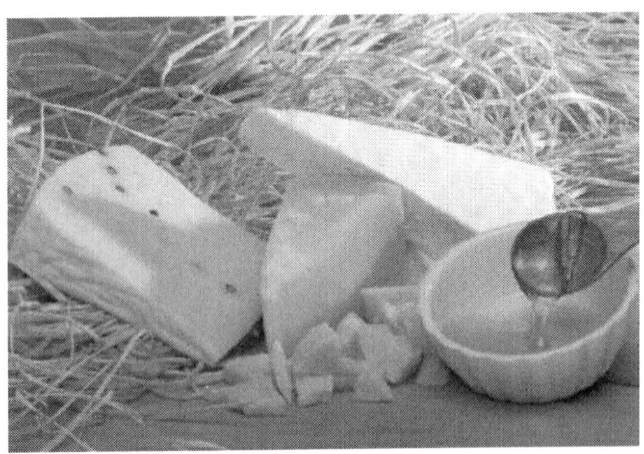

The Perfect Beginning: 2 lean sausages with 1 boiled egg (preferably soft boiled) and 1 kiwi fruit.

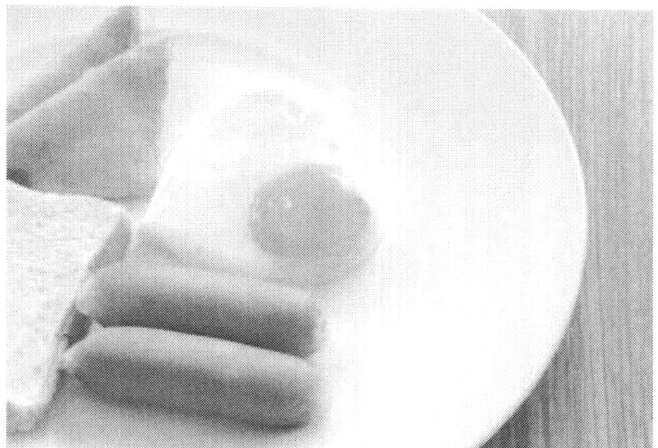

Lunch Choices:

Tuna and Bean Pita Wrap: ½ can of tuna, ¼ cup white beans, 1 teaspoon olive oil, 1 teaspoon lemon juice, 1 pita bread and 2 lettuce leaves. Use 1 cup of grapes as a side.

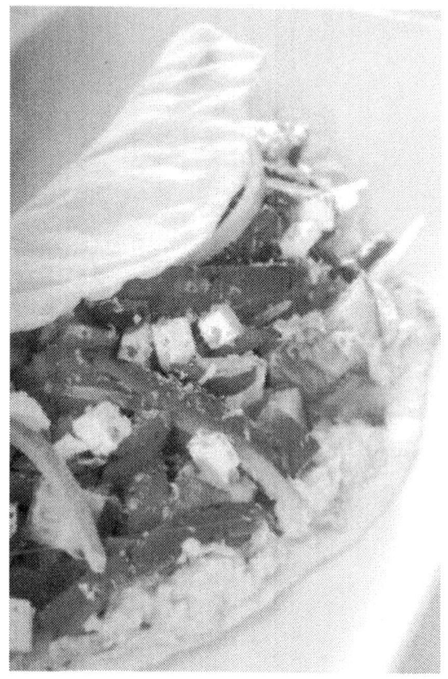

Egg and Vegetables Salad: 2 cups lettuce, 1 cup chopped vegetables of your choice, 1 hardboiled egg, 2 teaspoons almonds and 2 teaspoons raisins. Use 2 tablespoons balsamic vinegar as dressing.

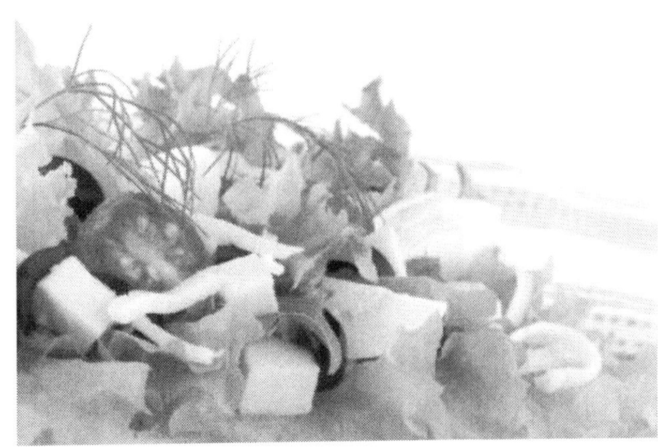

Vegetable Wrap: 1 pita bread topped with 20 grams feta cheese, 1 cup tomatoes, ¼ cup humus, 6 olives, 1 cup spinach, 1 teaspoon olive oil and 1 teaspoon lemon juice.

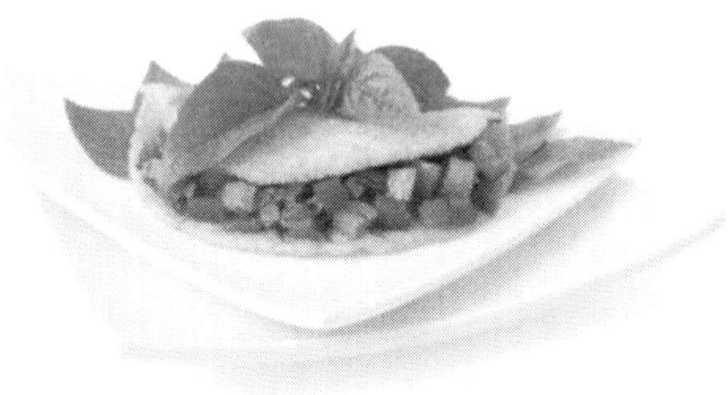

Lentil Soup with Seasoned Bread: 1 cup lentil soup. 1 pita bread topped with 1 teaspoon pesto sauce, 1 tablespoon sundried tomatoes and 2 tablespoons mozzarella cheese.

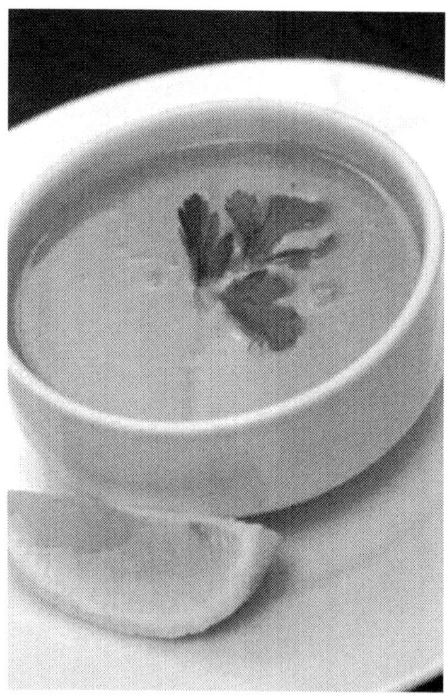

Tortilla Delights: 1 tortilla slice topped with 1/3 cup cheddar cheese and vegetables. Sauté ¼ cup green peppers, ¼ cup mushrooms and ¼ cup black beans in a little olive oil and add it to the top. Serve with ¼ of avocado.

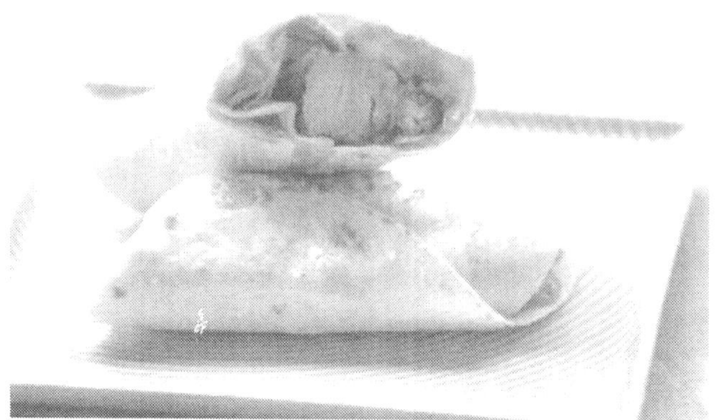

Tuna and Walnut Salad: 60 grams of tuna, 2 cups of spring greens, 3 tablespoons walnuts and 1 cup cherry tomatoes. Use 2 teaspoons balsamic vinegar as dressing.

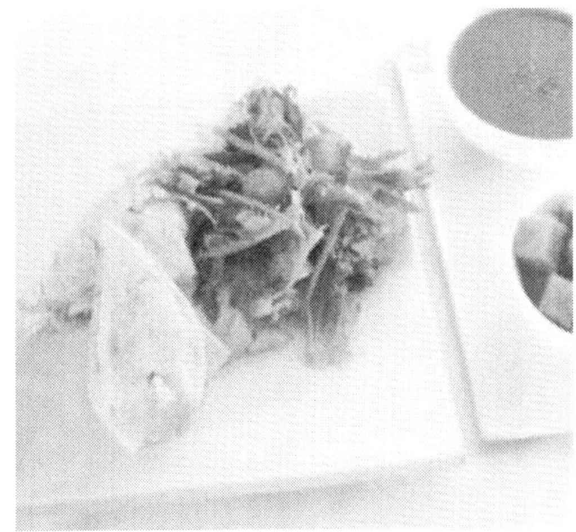

Sweet and Sour Sandwich: 2 slices of whole wheat bread, 1 teaspoon mustard paste, 5 slices of turkey, 1 pear sliced and 1 slice of cheese.

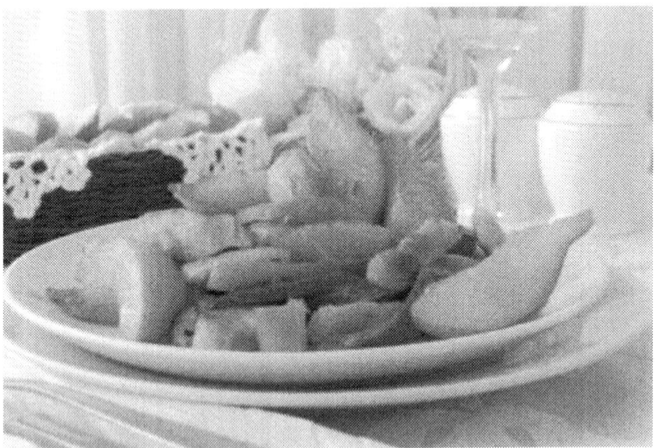

Black Bean Tortilla: 2 tortilla slices topped with ¾ cup black beans, ¼ avocado, 1 cup romaine lettuce and 2 tablespoons of salsa sauce.

Chicken Stuffed Pita: 1 pita bread topped with 1 cup diced and sautéed chicken, 2 tablespoons balsamic vinegar, ¼ cup chopped green onions, 1 stem of celery and 1 cup of salad greens.

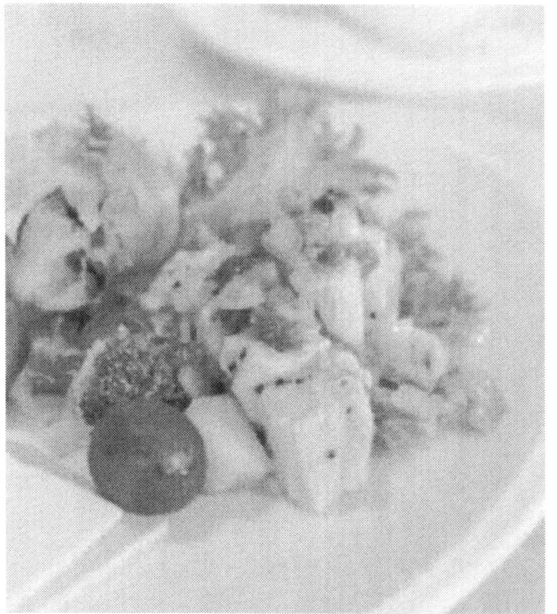

Dinner Choices:

Hot Black Bean Burger with Coleslaw Side: 1 black bean burger patty cooked with BBQ sauce for a spicy flavor. Use whole wheat bread to assemble the burger. Mix coleslaw made up of 1/3 cup of cabbage, 1/3 cup broccoli, 1.3 cup cauliflower, ½ cup carrots, 1 tablespoon apple cider vinegar and 2 tablespoons olive oil.

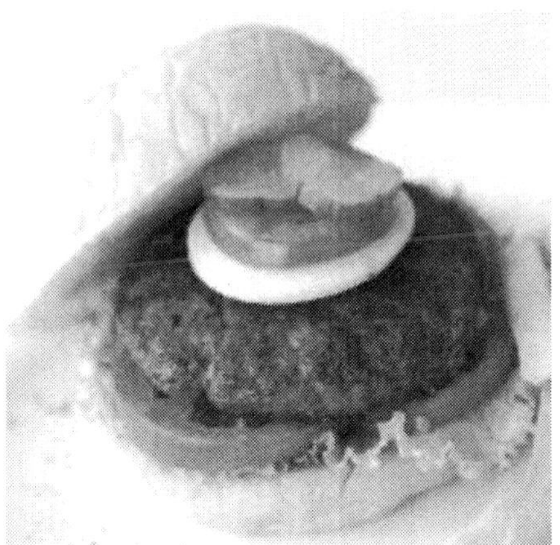

Shrimp Pasta: 1 cup whole wheat pasta of your choice, 40 grams of shrimp, 1 garlic clove, 1 cup zucchini, 2 tablespoons roughly chopped basil leaves and 1 tablespoon olive oil.

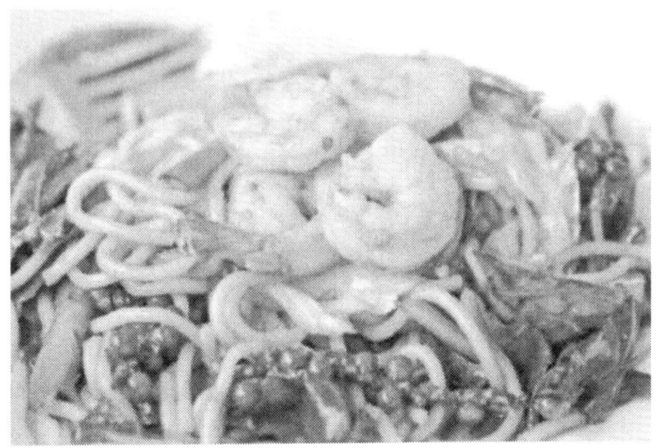

Spicy Peanut Chicken in Tortillas: 2 tortilla slices with 2/3 cup cubed and sautéed chicken, ¼ cup green onions, 2 tablespoons peanuts and 1 tablespoon hot sauce. Sauté 1/3 cup cabbage, 1/3 cup broccoli, 1/3 cup cauliflower and 1/3 cup carrot in another pan and add at the top.

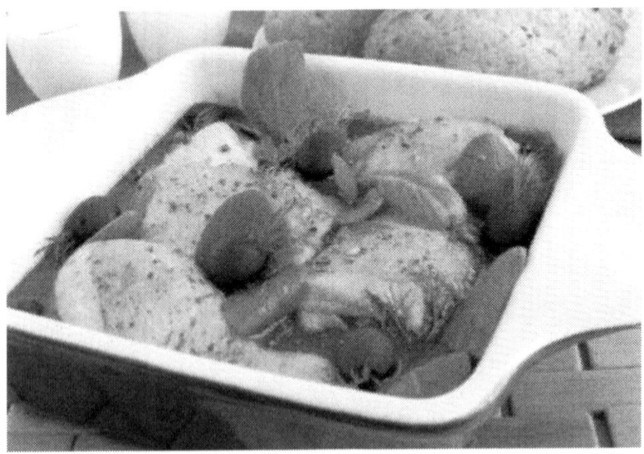

Marine Cuisine: 1 cup sushi, 1 tuna roll and 1 bowl of seaweed salad.

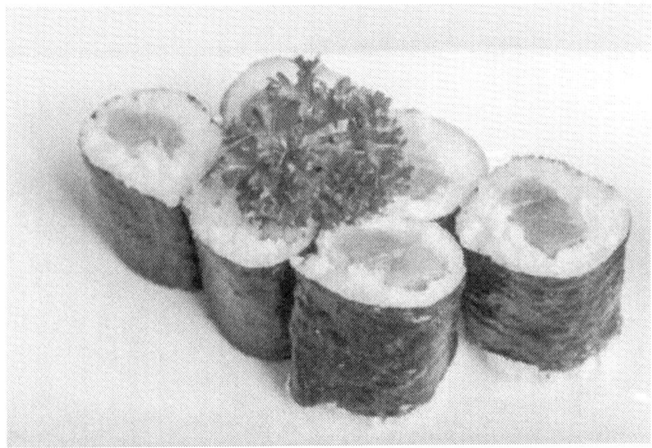

Bean Tortillas: 2 tortilla slices topped with ½ cup refried beans, sautéed vegetables and cilantro leaves. For sautéed vegetables, use 1 cup capsicum, ½ onion and 1 tablespoon olive oil.

Black Bean Tortilla Wraps: 2 tortilla slices topped with 1 cup zucchini, ½ cup black beans, and 1 teaspoon cumin sautéed in 2 teaspoons olive oil. Add cheese on the top and grill until cheese melts. Add 2 teaspoons of salsa on top.

Spicy Cheesy Tortilla with Salad Side: 8 tortilla chips, 2 tablespoons cheddar cheese, 2 tablespoons green onions and 1 cup vegetarian chili. For salad, use 2 cups mixed greens and 1 tablespoon Italian salad dressing.

Green Chicken with Goat Cheese: 100 grams chicken sautéed with 3 cups spinach, 2 tablespoons olive oil and 1 garlic clove. Place the mixture on a flatbread with 20 grams of goat cheese and grill to your desired color.

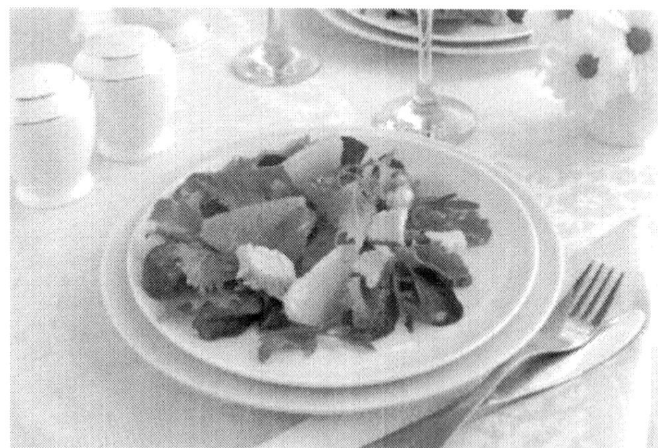

Shrimp with Fried Rice: Sauté 1 cup boiled brown rice, 1 tablespoon sesame oil, 1 tablespoon soy sauce, 1 garlic clove, 1 tablespoon ginger, 60 grams of cooked shrimp and 2 cups of Chinese cabbage.

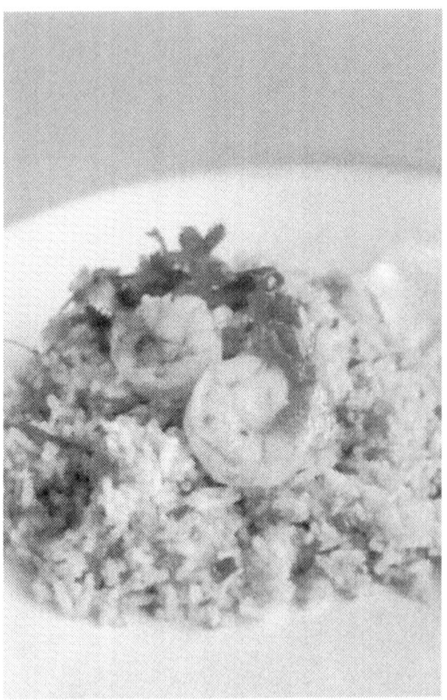

Meatless Pizza with Salad: 1 flat bread topped with 3 tablespoons spaghetti sauce, ½ cup artichoke, 2 tablespoons parmesan cheese and ¼ cup mozzarella cheese. Grill to your desired color. For salad, use 3 cups of mixed greens, 2 tablespoons pine nuts and 2 tablespoons of salad dressing.

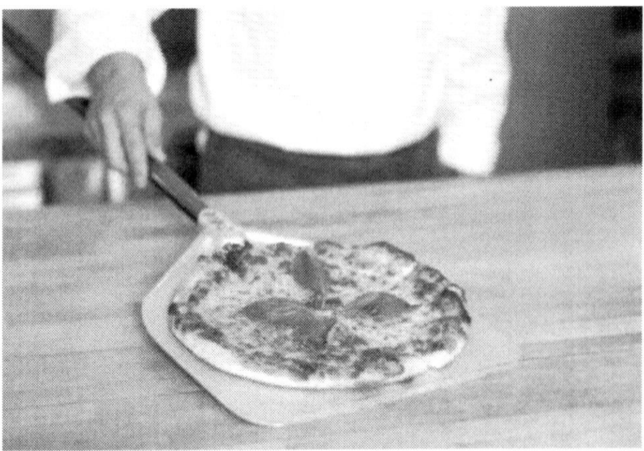

Stuffed Potato Pie: Use a baked potato for a base and top it with ½ cup turkey slices, 1 cup broccoli and ¼ cup cheddar cheese. Grill to desired color.

Sausage Pasta: Sauté 1 sliced sausage with 1 garlic clove, ½ cup mushrooms, ½ cup onions, ½ cup zucchini and ½ cup spaghetti sauce. Add it to ¾ cup pasta and top it with 1 tablespoon parmesan cheese.

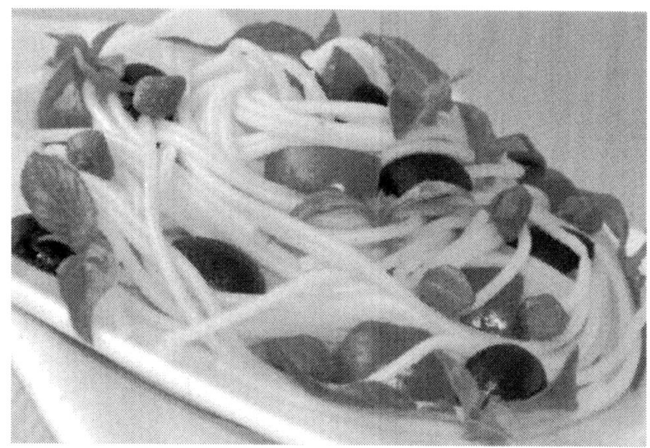

Spiced Chicken with Vegetable Rice: Cook 100 grams of chicken cubes with Cajun spices. Sauté 1 garlic clove, ½ cup chopped onions and 1 chopped bell pepper in 2 teaspoons oil. Add 2 tablespoons tomato sauce and 1 tablespoon Tabasco sauce. Add ¾ cup brown rice. Serve with chicken on the top!

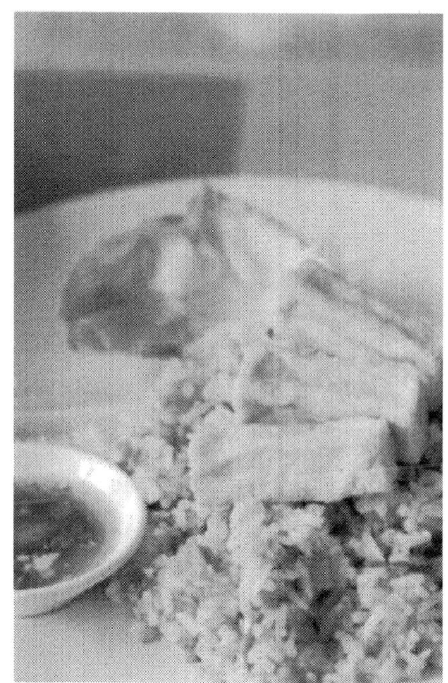

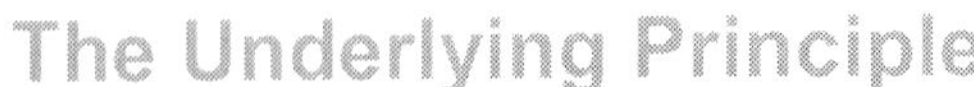

The Underlying Principle

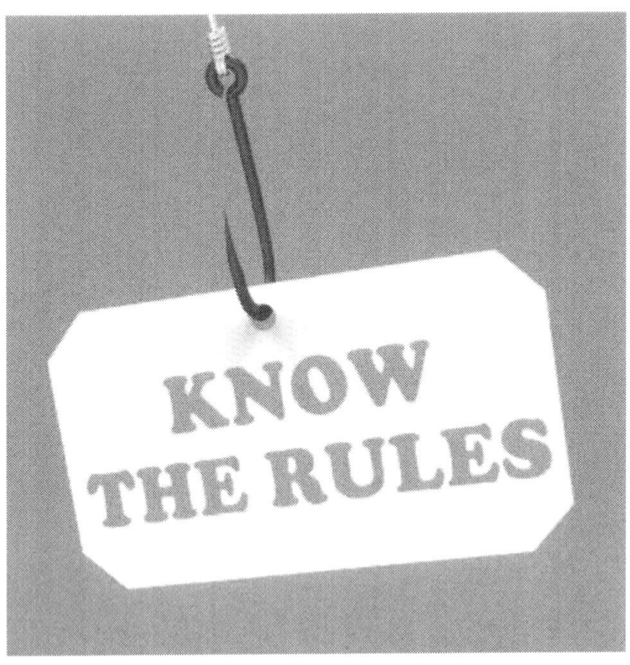

The Military Diet works by taking the chemical compositions of different foods into account. The individual food items are grouped in such a way that the aggregate effect of the combination helps you achieve your objectives. It encourages calorie burning and boosts the metabolic activity. So you are able to burn off the extra fats in your body quite effortlessly.

It does not compel you to go through strenuous exercise routines. It does, however, require you to indulge in adequate exercise on a daily basis. In effect, it needs lesser will power and commitment as compared to other starving diet plans.

Moreover, the diet plan is much cheaper compared to other alternatives. It does not incorporate the use of expensive pills or other chemicals which can cost you several dollars. It makes use of natural products that are known to complement each other. So you can achieve the desired level of fitness quickly, easily and readily!

The Military Diet plan yields results within a week. So naturally, it is your best resort if you would like to lose weight in an emergency. It has been narrated by the best of military professionals who used this diet plan to stay fit and to get back in shape after the break periods.

The Military Diet plan is known to be effective for all people in more or less the same way. There are no contraindications to the plan as the components of the regime are purely natural. All it needs is careful planning and execution to make sure the desired results can be achieved.

So do you really have it in you to make a positive change to yourself?!

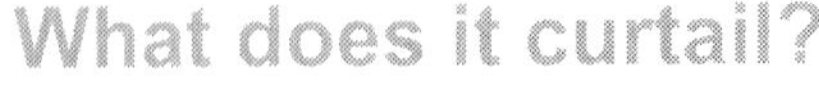

What does it curtail?

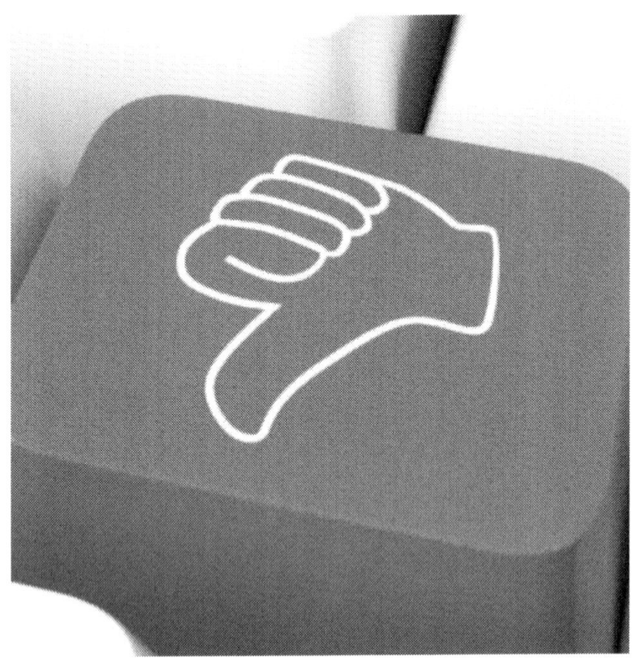

Generally, there are no such restrictions to your consumption when it comes to the Military Diet. It is a natural and well-proven way to achieve positive results. You do not need to deviate from your schedule much. The products you are required to consume are natural and safe in every possible way!

However, for best results, here are a few things that you need to keep in mind:

1. Size Does Not Matter. That is right! The serving size is not as pivotal to the diet plan as the number of calories that you consume. It is important that you do not deviate from the prescribed amount of calorie consumption. Otherwise, the overall impact of the routine will be lost.
   You need to consume a maximum of 1500 calories per day (adjust the figure according to your body weight). For males, you can add 100 calories more on this limit. This amount creates a calorie deficiency which in turn helps you lose excess body fat. Whether you are on the diet (3 days) or off it (4 days), the total number of calories you consume in a day should be equivalent to the mentioned amount.
   You can substitute the prescribed foods according to your personal preferences. However, make sure the aggregate number of calories per day remains the same. Use alternative food choices intelligently to ensure you are steadily moving towards the desired goals.
2. Restrict Sugar Intake. It is best if you quit sugar altogether! Given the health problems associated with the use of sugars, it is best if the leave this product in entirety.

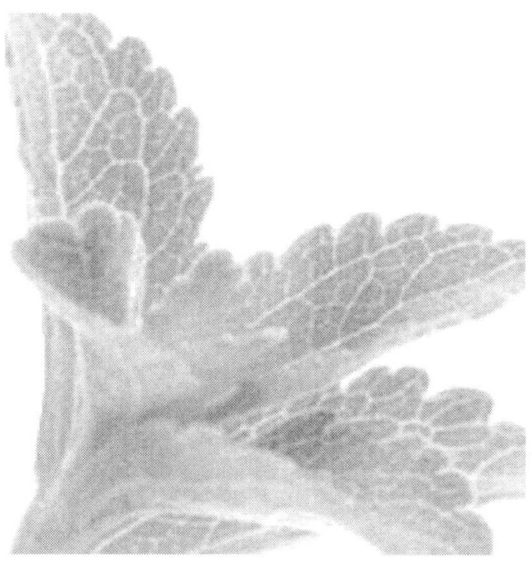

However, if you are one of those who cannot survive without some sweetness in life, use natural sweeteners like Stevia instead. On the same note, don't use artificial sweeteners either because they work in more or less the same way as refined sugars. Artificial sugars are known to impact your health negatively. Stevia, therefore, is the only natural sweetener that you can use while on the Military Diet or otherwise!

3. Snacking is Inappropriate. The idea behind the Military Diet is to restrict you to a diet of 1500 calories or so per day! It is considered normal to feel slightly hungry during the long hours after lunch. However, if you've survived this time well, it will automatically open the doors of success for you!

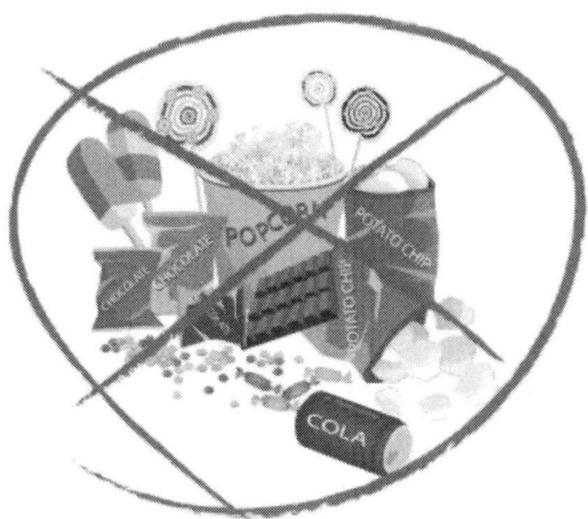

If you can absolutely not control your hunger pangs and have no leftovers from your latest meal to nibble on, the next best option is to go for healthy snacks.

Though do keep in mind that this will impact the total number of calorie intake so you will need to adjust an equivalent amount of calories from your dinner!
The general rule of thumb says avoid snacks. But if you really must, opt for the healthy ones only!

4. Coffee – To Drink or Not? It is one of the biggest concerns for Military Diet followers everywhere. Most people cannot survive without their daily intake of caffeine. The good news is you do not need to sacrifice this energy booster. The only thing you need to keep in mind is to adjust the calories counter with every cup of coffee that you consume.

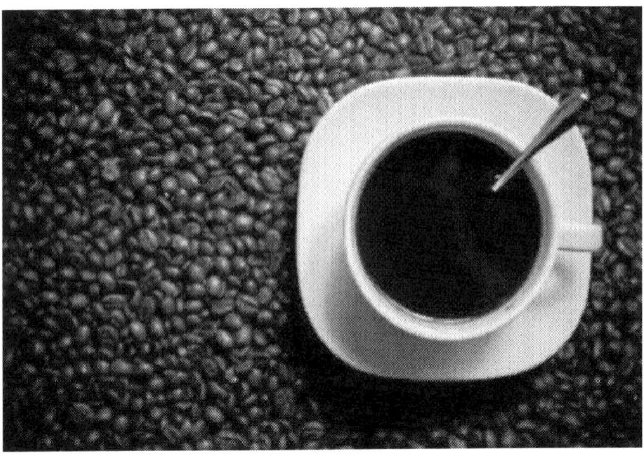

Black, sugar-free and cream-free coffee or tea is worth roughly 10 calories. So with every cup you consume, remember to take down an equivalent number of calories from your day's intake.
For those who do not like coffee, it is not as though it is an absolutely essential part of the diet plan. You can substitute it with green tea or other similar beverages if you would like. The idea behind coffee usage is that it stimulates the metabolic activity slightly. You can achieve the same results while drinking green tea and other similar drinks!

Conclusion

To sum it all up, the Military Diet is the surest way to reduce the inches, decrease the pounds and also attain internal fitness – all in one! It is an easy-to-follow routine that is not only natural but also allows you to take four days off the plan after every three days! It gets easier after the first day!

Moreover, the military men used it with great success! When it worked for them, it will surely work for the average individual! There are quite a few success stories circulating that talk about the impressive success ratios attached with the Military Diet. All the more reason to try out the Military Diet plan and savor the sweet sense of victory!

So if you are looking for a quick way to fit into a dress or to show off a picture-perfect body this season, the Military Diet plan is the course to pursue. It is a natural plan of action that compels you to restrict your calorie intake for greater gains.

You can enjoy your favorite foods, substitute those that do not agree with your taste buds and basically enjoy every delicacy there is! At the same time, you can see noticeable results that keep you motivated towards the plan!

And once you have achieved the results you have yearned for, don't forget to share your success stories for the world to know that the Military Diet plan works – for everyone!

We wish you all the best for your fitness endeavors and sincerely hope you will be able to attain your objectives. After all, there is no reason why it should not!

Printed in Great Britain
by Amazon